Vibrant at Any Age

*A guide to renew your life and become
vigorous, healthy, and happy*

Dr. Josefina Monasterio

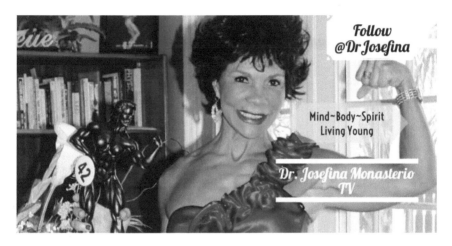

Life Coach, Bodybuilder, and TV Host

Printed in the United States of America

ISBN-13: 978-1539765806
ISBN-10: 1539765806

Pictures are in the public domain or labeled for reuse.

Vibrant at Any Age series

Book One: Vibrant at Any Age: A guide to renew your life and become vigorous, healthy, and happy

Book Two: Vibrant at Any Age: Live longer and useful all the days of your life

You can reach Dr. Josefina at DrJosefina@att.net

Website: www.DrJosefina.com
Facebook: www.facebook.com/drjosefina
Twitter: www.twitter.com/drjosefina
YouTube: www.youtube.com/drjosefina

I can't say enough about this inspirational book, I could not put it down. I feel so empowered and positive, like I can do ANYTHING! Dr. Josefina is an amazing ageless woman who has brought life to others in a healthy positive way. Love her attitude. We all need to follow her ways. I can't wait for Dr. Josefina's other books! If you haven't purchased, you need to! P.V.

Thanks for empowering us with the knowledge we need to live long and healthy lives. I'm reading on my way to church and I'm driving everyone crazy reading out loud every other paragraph! A.D.

Loved your book, so inspirational and empowering. I cannot stop reading it, especially about cutting out negative people from our lives. I will focus and think of it when I'm at work with negative coworkers. C.Q.

Wonderful insights and full of easy, positive methods to gain back your sense of direction and self. Dr. Josefina has a contagious attitude of hope and practical techniques that equip anyone, at any age, to learn happier life skills. E.M.

Dr. Josefina's book is amazing! It's excellent for any age or stage of life. She provides practical and easy to follow advice on developing a strong body and mind. It's uplifting, positive, and empowering! K.C.

The word "holistic" encompasses the health of our whole being: body, mind, and spirit. This book reflects just such an achievement in the life of the author. With the authority of a life lived she lays out how to achieve a unified self, thereby optimizing physical health, mental-emotional stability, and spiritual insight. Well worth reading. R.R.

Contents

Preface

What inspired me to write this book? Invariably, when I am at the gym, at shows, or just going about my business, people would come up and ask how old I am. When I tell them that I am 70 years old, they invariably exclaim something like, "Look at her, and we can hardly walk." They would go on to tell me how inspirational I am. Or they would ask, "Do you have a book so I can learn how to become like you?"

So that's why I am writing this book: to share, empower, and inspire others to embrace their unlimited potential. By developing healthy habits you also can enjoy a life of health, energy, and meaning.

Introduction

Earth no longer is flat as once believed. Likewise is it crucial to believe the new paradigm and change our belief system derived from our experience with aging. Aging has a negative connotation; it is not a disease. It is not a time to feel useless, sit in a corner, and watch the world alive around us.

My work is to change that ugly image; it is old age thinking. I want you to make the connection that by changing several lifestyle habits you can sit in the driver's seat towards a healthier and younger you. By making conscious choices you take responsibility to evolve your spirit, maintain a healthy physical body—biological machine—and improve your emotional health and mental attitude towards life.

I have found that successful people powerfully commit to achieving the changes they want. My wish for you, dear reader, is to muster the inspiration, determination, discipline, and energy to make those changes that will propel you to your next level.

You will be encouraged to reinvent yourself as you feel in your gut that your ongoing development and perfectioning is working. You will discover that your chronological age has nothing to do with your physical age, that your life is not over because age has a number attached to it. You will *feel* in control of your physical, mental, and spiritual health because you will *be* in control.

I know from experience with my clients and myself that following these lifestyle changes will transform you into an enthusiastic and awesome person. You will develop a profound self-respect, increase your energy, and optimize your health. You will feel and be invincible. Wow! How's that for a goal?

My Story

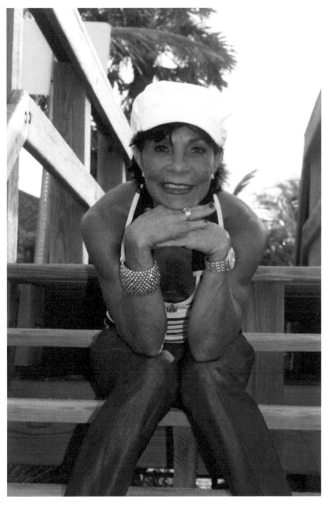

I have written about myself because we teach by our lives, by what we do, and not so much by what we say. And I am foremost a teacher, sharing how to become all you are capable of becoming.

• • •

I was born in the small town Punta de Mata in the state of Monagas, Venezuela. I lived a life of poverty of things, but not a scarcity of dreams.

I fondly remember happy memories of my childhood, especially with my father. Although he deserted the family when I was five, I knew he loved me. My mom was only a teenager when my grandmother took in my brother and me and raised us. What a model of a hard worker she was, never complaining as she shouldered the almost impossible task of keeping a roof over our head and food on the table. But that didn't impoverish her attitude. She never, ever told me I could not do something.

I looked at my grim life and decided this would not be my future. We were financially poor; there was no fortune to inherit. I walked two miles to school, often with just a chunk of bread for lunch. Thank God we wore school uniforms because I had only one dress.

But I knew that real richness was in my mind. I knew early on that the best route to get what I wanted lay through education. My childhood instilled and confirmed these beliefs that remained and grew throughout my life.

You always have your dreams

One of my greatest blessings has been my positive attitude, how I perceive the world regardless of what it's like around me. As a young girl I had a sense of hope that exciting events awaited me. Although of lowly beginning, I had my dreams, goals, and hopes for a brighter, greater future.

I worked hard and was fortunate to have wonderful teachers who made a difference in my life. I remember lying in the grass at night, and as the stars came out, I dreamed. I saw my future. I knew then that I would reach the stars. I

4

visualized myself in the USA or Germany going to school, getting my Masters Degree, a dream that did not fade as it continued to energize me to keep on with my studies. This despite the circumstances and reality around me that cried, *No, you can't! You will have nothing.* It's not true. You always have your dreams—if you dare dream them.

School

During my school years my teachers mentored, supported, and encouraged my dreams and goals.

My first degree was from Escuela Normal Miguel Antonio Caro as an elementary school teacher. My first job after graduating was teaching sixth grade. After my first year one of the teachers encouraged me to go beyond teaching at the elementary school level, and so I returned to school to get a degree that would allow me to teach in high school, a decision that changed the course of my life. In particular, fellow teacher Dario Silva awakened in me the belief that I could do whatever I set my mind to do.

It was not only her encouragement that I remember but also how she helped make it happen. She encouraged me to focus on physical education (PE) and recommended me for a position as a PE teacher, making more money, and with flexible hours so I could pursue my education. Then she used her influence to get me one of the scarce openings at the Instituto Pedagogico de Caracas, Venezuela, where I received my second college degree in physical education. I excelled at sports from an early age, and in time became an excellent runner and gymnast, which is why I majored in physical education.

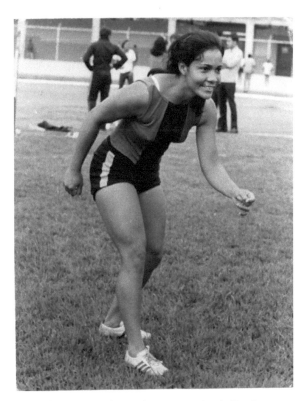

All the while I continued to teach full time to help my mother and pay for my expenses.

I continued to meet the most wonderful teachers. They became my inspiration because they had accomplished what I wanted to do. Their reality became my vision: continue pursuing higher education.

• • •

The challenge was to go overseas to achieve what they had done. But I needed the money to make my vision a reality. Not having it didn't discourage me; my dreams were my currency. I continued seeing myself reach my dreams. Each evening after training I would lie down on the grass and visualize myself reaching my dream. It was then that I discovered the power of the subconscious mind. Thoughts would rise to my conscious mind regarding what I should do to accomplish my goal. The discovery of how the subconscious and conscious minds work together energized me to follow and act on my inner guidance.

I also discovered its best not to share my goals with people who haven't been there and lack vision. They are the ones who tell you that you can't.

A scholarship

One of these thoughts I received was to apply for a scholarship, make appointments with people who can help, show them my credentials and why I deserve it. My friends and mentors also encouraged my thinking and urged me to pursue my education and seek scholarships. Following my vision was not easy with my days often starting at 5 AM waiting for the Minister of Education's early arrival. I thought, *Others want these scholarships so do something different. I need to see him to prove myself.*

Well, I won the award! My vision and diligence paid off. I now had a choice between Europe and the United States. Friends urged me to choose the United States. "Go to Boston for the best education," they told me, "and to California or Florida for the best weather."

Boston to Vero Beach, Florida

I chose Boston University for my Master's Degree in education. I am so grateful that I made this decision. It greatly broadened my experience by mastering English, learning how others live, and seeing things through their eyes. Being around Harvard University and the Massachusetts Institute of

Technology was intellectually challenging, but it fostered flexibility and creative thinking.

After receiving my degree, my God-given gifts made room for me, especially Spanish. Along with Spanish, I taught science, biology, and health at Cambridge High School. The sizeable Spanish-speaking population from Nicaragua, Santo Domingo, and San Salvador enabled me to serve as a teacher-advisor. I also had a television program reporting on consumer affairs, broadcast in English and Spanish. I organized a nutrition and fitness club for teenagers. We worked out three mornings a week at seven in the morning—even when the weather was below zero. Brrr! Enough with the cold already!

• • •

This was my life until I perceived it was time to move on. I had bought a home in Vero Beach and I would fly south during school breaks every eight weeks or so. While I loved almost everything about New England, the frigid exception was the ice-block winter; I could no longer stand the cold.

Originally, I had planned to take a year's leave from work. It so happened that the Vero Beach campus of the community college was nearby. When I saw the advertisement for an academic advisor, I applied, was hired, and my life shifted fully to Vero Beach.

I found advising college students quite different than struggling with high school teenagers. The older students wanted help; with them I could make a difference. Reaching teenagers is very difficult because their home life affects their self-esteem. I provided a learning environment that encouraged their self-esteem and inspired their imagination to become all that they are capable of becoming, to draw on their courage to follow their dreams. Teens are at that stage of development where they hate you for what you are, and hate themselves for what they are not. I still love them, and they love me back, and I continue to hear from them.

By contrast, older learners have purpose and motivation to improve their lives. That is the difference.

I love working with both.

• • •

I continued the dream in Vero Beach that began in Boston where I had been a TV Host. I created my own TV show called *Empowerment with Dr. Josefina*. It leveraged my ability to empower others by sharing with a wider audience the principles by which anyone can be vibrant, successful, and healthy.

A surprise awaited me, a life-changing event that *seemed to happen* of its own accord, that some might say mere coincidence, but it is not so. To paraphrase Einstein, *God doesn't play dice with your life.*

I *chanced* to meet Steve, who saw in me the potential to become an outstanding bodybuilder, muscled and strong. What, me! Wondering how this drama could play out, I told Steve, "I don't have a clue how to go about it." He said the magic words, "I will help you." Then I knew this was my new direction. While many are quick to tell you what they see is best for you, few are willing to help you achieve it. That's what set Steve apart. Isn't life an adventure?

I began bodybuilding at age 59. (It's *never* too late to change where you are going.) It was beautiful how Steve didn't see age; he saw potential. What a blessing. He took me under his wings, trained me, and in just six months I entered

9

my first bodybuilding show—and I won first place! My fledgling wings spread wide as I soared to the skies!

I've been at it now for 11 years, thrilled with winning the *Masters Bodybuilding* competition and lauded as *Best Female Bodybuilder* at many other events. I mention these accolades to encourage you. They show what vision, determination, and attitude can accomplish in your life.

Bodybuilding changed my life. It solidified my health and slowed down the aging process, adding years to my life. It formed a body powerful and resilient with increased muscle mass and bone density. Result: I feel terrific!

People feel the passion and energy I bring to the sport of bodybuilding when they see me posing.

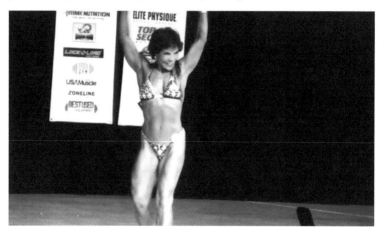

Many have gratefully told me that seeing inspired them to either compete or seriously take care of their bodies. Such unexpected confirmation that you have followed the plan for your life is thrilling!

Do what you love—always!

The power of never giving up

Another of my dreams was to get my doctorate degree (PhD). I had wanted to do it in Boston where the school system in which I taught offered the faculty free tuition to continue their education. It was a splendid opportunity, but my children were too young. It forced the decision to be a mom and pursue my dream later. Right choice; glad I made it.

By the time the children were in first and second grade I could no longer endure the eternally long, dreary, and cold Boston winters. That's it! I'm moving to Vero Beach, Florida. Although no schools in the area offered a PhD program, it did not occur to me that I would not achieve my goal. I knew it would happen; I just didn't know how.

Then I got a job at the satellite campus of Barry University as an Academic Adviser. I shared with my director, Dr. Beverly Whitely, my desire to continue my education. She told me she received her degree from Nova University, which I could do remotely from Vero Beach. I enrolled, she mentored me, and I graduated with my doctorate degree.

Here's the takeaway from my experience: know what you want and trust with steadfast faith that you will achieve it.

Choose Who You Want to Be

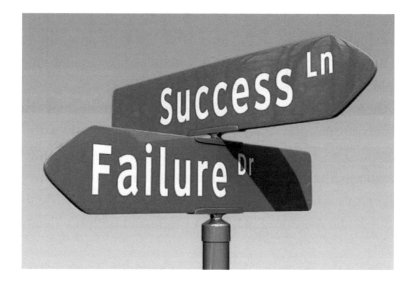

Successful Aging

While we can't choose how long we live, we can determine how well we do it. To achieve this we must take responsibility for our choices in each area of our lives.

Many people believe that growing older means sickness, medications, feebleness, and lack of purpose. Life is over! Some of the words used to describe older people are bitter, mean, sour, boring, dull, slow and depressing. How sad to look forward to losing your physical independence and burdening others with your ill health, not to mention being set aside because you are useless. No wonder people are terrified of getting old.

The older you get, the better you should feel, like a wine that has aged. But aging successfully requires a choice. To me successful aging means feeling happy with your health, pleased with your body, satisfied with your energy level, and enjoying activities you love. It happens because you take care of your body *every single day*. You do it by good nutrition, portion control, daily exercise, sleeping well, stress-free relaxation, reflective meditation, and heartfelt prayer.

Appreciating the beauty around us is crucial to successfully aging. Perhaps, like me, you would enjoy rising at 4 AM and going for a walk or run, with a companion or alone, feeling the soft and enchanting hours of the day's beginning as the stars and planets linger in their majesty and the silvery moonlight enthralls you. The sounds of creation surround you as the birds welcome the new day. And there you are taking it all in. How I do it may not appeal to everyone, but however you do it, consciously appreciating the beauty around you slows down the aging process.

Another crucial aspect of successful aging is a sense of purpose. You do that by re-creating yourself. Every ten years is my number. Choose a number that fits you. Numbers define career stages as you move into new positions and challenges, whether it be a mother, teacher, doctor, nurse, or banker. Then one day, POW! You're just an "old retired person." Of course that will do a job on your self-image and self-esteem—unless you reinvent yourself.

Find a new focus in your life, and then follow the way that achieves it. Remember, while purpose changes with time, its form and essence remain the same. You did it before; you can do it again. Your life will gain a new reason for being, along with the excitement, energy, and joy of being alive. Your attitude about life and about yourself will reach a new height. As you renew your thinking and make your thoughts loving, positive, and constructive, you will feel powerful, better than ever, grateful to live joyfully.

Another key for successful aging is ATTITUDE. Delighting to see what unfolds day-by-day makes enthusiasm a way of life. You find yourself associating with energetic, optimistic, passionate, healthy, and happy people who encourage one other. Surround yourself with them. They know that life is a self-fulfilling prophesy, that we don't always get what we want, but we do get what we expect. They expect the best.

Use affirmations daily to empower yourself. We become what we envision, reflect on, and tell ourselves, whether good or bad.

Make enthusiasm a way of life, be passionate about every single day, and see your life come alive. Be your own cheerleader.

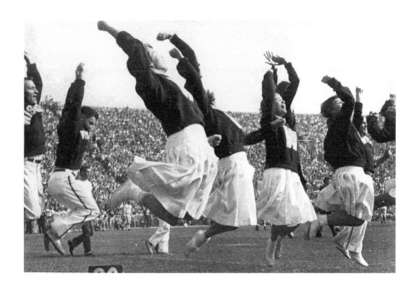

Laugh a lot. Laughter benefits our physiology, our health in every area. "A merry heart does good like a medicine." It is a tranquilizer without side effects. Hmm, I feel better already.

Above all, be thankful and grateful for the privilege of one more day, one more chance to express yourself and bless others.

The Chapter of Hope

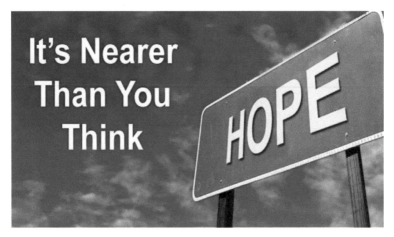

Hope is like an insurance policy. When we're feeling discouraged, down and out, we draw upon our policy of hope and our spirit revives. But it's more than a reservoir of strength, it is *knowing* that things will get better. It fuels us with high octane power to keep going and never give up.

Where does this hope come from? I believe it is innate; we are born with the instinct to believe the invisible dream—unseen by our mortal eyes, but not to the eyes of spirit.

How hope helped me

I always knew that by expecting the best and acting on my vision that the things I wanted would happen, and most of the time they would be better than I expected.

Hope kept me alive no matter what was going on around me and happening to me. It kept me on my path, thereby enabling me to take advantage of the opportunities life brought my way.

How do you know you have hope?

Hope gives you joy. Joy is the shortcut of assessing the hope that lies within you. More particularly:

- You believe and trust that your vision will come to pass. It is the strong sense that what you want will happen and things will turn out for the best.

- Hope fuels optimism, along with faith and love.

- Hope expects the desire of your heart to manifest, thereby giving you a reason to live. It gives you a future. Without hope, you no longer have a reason for your life. You give up as you die in spirit.

- Hope fills you with peace and joy.

- Hope makes you feel secure.

- Hope doesn't wear out (although it may grow thin at times ☺); it is untiring.

- Hope keeps you going during times of darkness and adversity.

- Hope comes from developing and cultivating your spiritual nature, essential to overcoming the challenges that life presents. Hope gives you the patience to endure them.

- Hope empowers you because you believe you can. And you know what? YES, YOU CAN!

Setting Goals

You first need to know where you are going before you can get there. Makes sense, doesn't it? So how do you do this?

- Ask yourself, *What do I want?* From the ocean of possibilities, which will you choose and focus on?
- Then believe your goal will happen. This is the faith element. Others have achieved similar goals, so ask yourself, *Why not me?*
- Your goal then imprints on your subconscious as you reflect on it and come to believe you are worthy of it. This is crucial: your spirit loves and nurtures you as the most loving parent you can image. Spirit finds no fault with you. She nourishes your dreams and aspirations and works behind the scenes to make them happen.

Here's how I brought into being one of my goals.

I was determined to not only leave my life of poverty in Venezuela but also excel by coming to the United States. I didn't know how I would do it, only that I would surely do it.

Then the creative part of my mind began telling me: Talk to the Minister of Education, speak with that person, make this phone call, and so on. I began following my intuition, which strengthened my connection to spirit.

No matter how bad things are, they don't have to change your goal, the dream of where you want to go.

Victor Frankel believed he would survive the Nazi concentration camp. His goal? Get out alive and share what he experienced with the world. And that's what he did.

You can be in horrible circumstances, yet they are your passport out of them, unlikely as it seems. The experience will elevate you to a higher place — provided you have hope, you have a dream, you have a goal, you have a passion—and you believe it is possible. Then that is exactly what will happen.

Attitude

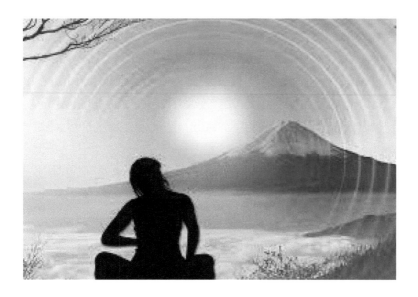

After your dream comes attitude. Your attitude determines your success and failure in life. For example, if everything stinks, your life will smell. On the other hand, while a rose has its thorns, it still smells sweet.

Life gives you back what you put out to others. Not only does it add wonderful relationships but also the vibrancy of living. Your success and failure in whatever you do is based on your relationship with others. When people see you, how do they greet you and treat you? Do they run away? *Oh God, I don't want to talk to him!* Or, *Oh Josefina, how great to see you!*

If you have a good attitude toward life, it will compensate you for its difficulties and challenges. Some people become jaded in their sense of life, of hope, of what they can do; they do not let themselves believe they can successfully deal with life's issues. Someone puts them into an age category and tells them they can't do this, and you know what? They can't.

A good attitude doesn't mean your life is perfect. It means you control how you react to its events. You are the thermostat and not the thermometer.

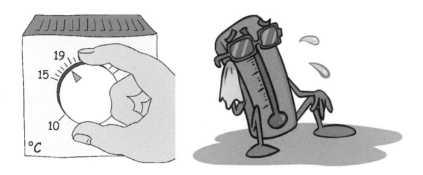

How I maintain a good attitude

I developed an awareness of my attitude and took steps if it wasn't where it should be. For example, when raising my kids I'd stay in my room if I had a bad day.

I check that my attitude is positive whenever I leave home. I do not have the right to be nasty, mean, miserable, and ugly to others. Our job is to bring joy, happiness, and hope. Especially these days, people need to have the hope you'll share. Attitude determines how you feel about yourself, your self-esteem, your self-image—and how you feel about others.

If I have a negative attitude, my goals will fail. No one will help me with them. By contrast, with a good attitude everywhere I go people go out of their way to help me. Why? I'm *always* nice to others. As a result, when I need help, no problem because I've made an investment in other people. Be nice! Be nice! It's called love in action.

I go to the supermarket and occasionally I am annoyed. I just want to get my potatoes and leave, yet workers come over and ask, "Are you finding everything okay? Is there anything I can help you with?" And I think to myself, "Why don't they go help that lady?" My life-force has drawn them without them being aware. They want to be around someone positive, happy, and vibrant for a few moments. I recognize immediately that it's not accidental. My annoyance leaves and I'm nice, I'm nice.

Another example of keeping a good attitude: I remember distinctly being in a bodybuilding competition in which I refused to allow anxiety or anything negative decide my attitude. The result? The competitive pressure propelled, energized, and focused my attitude on achieving success.

Where my attitude came from

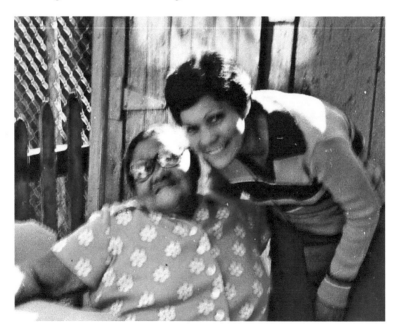

My grandmother was my foundation, my symbol of strength and power. She never complained despite being a single woman raising me, my brother, and the child of a mother who rejected her. We learned to take responsibility by how she lived. It is where I learned discipline, determination, and attitude.

She never told me I couldn't do something. She let me have my dreams, like when I decided the impossible: attend school overseas in the United States.

Some people are born with a good attitude and some are born without it. It is similar to being a leader; you are either a born leader or you acquire it through determination, discipline, and education because you have something to say and you want to lead people into a way of life.

Fortunately, I was born with a joyful attitude. It is innate. It's one of my greatest gifts. My attitude reflects my joy, which comes from my spirit.

My mom used to say to me, *You think that life is a bowl of roses*. And it was. I was always singing, dreaming, and happy. I never lost the child in me. Sometimes we lose that child. We lose the laughter, sense of humor, and joy as we grow up. We lose it all.

But I kept it. I knew there's a better way whatever happened to me. When you choose life, it works beautifully.

Life has its own programming and it's going to work as long as you don't fight it.

Here's an example: When writing this book, my computer broke and I had to send it out for repair. Here I was waiting for my writing partner to come and I had no computer. What was I to do? No problem; I went with what life had prepared. I said, Richard, the computer broke. Where do we go from here?

When we begin trusting life and how it *always* works out, life becomes easier and happier.

Here's how you can identify a positive attitude. Regardless of your circumstances—what happens to you, how old you are, and so on—you always see the possibilities. How I am now is not where I will end up. Some of us have the vision and skill to see our lives in the future. You know that who I am now is not what I am all about. You refuse to give up becoming all you are capable of being.

I grew up in a small town in Venezuela. My aunt Dilia had ten children, each with a different dad. As a child and a teenager I looked at that scenario and said to myself, *That is not for me!* People want to blame everything on something or someone else: *I was born into it; I didn't have the money*, and so on. Don't do it. Rather, look at your life and say, *This is not what I want to do with my life.* That's what I did. Even at a young age I had the attitude that I didn't want my family to have a different father for each child.

Forgive yourself

I was working with a client and we talked about forgiving her bad feelings toward her brother. This may shock you, but she said to me, *Josefina, if I forgive him who will I hate?* Ugh! Some people refuse to forgive because they need someone to hate; they feel alive this way.

Forgiveness is the key to happiness. You will not be content until you forgive. The negative energy of your emotions imprisons you. Forgiving others opens the cell door and you walk out a free person. Although bad feelings do leave when you forgive another, you must replace them with the opposite; otherwise, they will return.

> My family almost poisoned me about my dad. If I had listened, I would have believed that Josefina is unlovable because my father left me. Fortunately, I recalled fond memories of him lovingly tossing me in the air—my antidote to the poison I had begun to drink.

Here's a way to go about removing the poison of a nurtured grudge. Quiet yourself, sit down, and reflect on the negative experience—as I did with my dad. It liberated me and it will free you as well. Get a piece of paper and write down where the beliefs you bought into came from, the ones that define who you are. Then decide what is true. Now you'll know what to stop believing and begin living free.

It takes commitment to free yourself from believing error about who you are. Forgiveness follows when you do so. You become the person you want to be, an unstoppable success in life, always growing. You feel good about yourself; you are glad to be you; you like who you are. That's being rich; that's having true wealth.

Have I wronged others?

> When your life is sweet, it does not result from happenstance, but by a life aligned with that which is right.

Have I wronged others? Think deeply; it will come to you. Immediately correct what you did, even if it happened years ago or the person has died. How do you do this?

Meditate to reach a higher level of consciousness. Speak to the person and say, *I'm sorry for hurting you.* Because spirit communicates by its own circuits, it doesn't matter if you cannot actually reach the person. Your sincere repentance gets through and it frees you. However, if the person is available, apologize face-to-face or by phone.

If you cheated and money was involved, make restitution. Restore what you took unfairly. The money is not yours to use; you got it unjustly. If that person is unavailable, take that money and do good to others with it.

And if money was not involved, be inspired how to make right that which is wrong. It will not only free you but the other person as well if he or she is feeling bad to you.

After you have cleared the past and the guilt that accompanies wrongdoing, whenever you do something that makes you feel guilty, be sure it's wrong according to your innermost being, not because of what others say. If indeed you've done harm, ask yourself, *How can I make it right?* Do so and don't do it again.

What are the steps to develop a positive attitude?

What if you're not born with a good attitude and don't know how to acquire it?

1. First, decide that I want my life to be better. I deserve my life to be better. I deserve to be successful. It doesn't make a difference whether you wash dishes or clean house. Success comes from how happy you feel doing whatever it is you are doing.

2. Then refuse to allow circumstances, parents, teachers, church, and so on, tell you that you're no good.

    Be aware that others may have a plan for you; don't buy into it. People are quick to tell you how to run your life. Although their intentions may be good, no one knows what's best for you; only you do. But you must have the guts, audacity, and attitude to say, *Thank you, but no thanks*. And be nice about it.

3. A good attitude derives from the relationship you have with yourself. Feeling bad about yourself is self-destructive in many ways, such as the out-of-control use of drugs, alcohol, sex, and food. A bad attitude harms your health.

    If this describes you, it is essential to change how you feel about yourself. No one is your best friend but you. Learn to like yourself and become your best friend. When you work on this with determination, discipline, and commitment, things change. Count on it!

4. When something disturbs you, immediately make sure your attitude is under control. Do not allow the negative energy of other people or situation to find a resting place.

You can say something like, *I release you*, and allow the thought or emotion to pass away.

5. Practice. The more you practice being positive, the stronger you become. Like everything in life, when you train every day, whether it's your physical muscles, spiritual muscles, or attitude muscles, your attitude keeps growing, and growing, and growing. Like Jack and the beanstalk, cultivate your tiny seedling and it can't help but become a high climbing vine.

The flipside of practice is perseverance. In other words, don't give up! Life is on your side.

Now that I have a good attitude, what next?

Your joy is your strength as energy infuses you with vigor. Happiness confirms that you are living the life you should. It proclaims *Heaven approves of how I am living!*

Once you have a good attitude and encounter issues with parents, those you love, strangers—everyone—you are now equipped to handle them.

I was in Miami visiting my friend, and she said, "Let's go to the gym." When I went to register myself as a guest, the guy at the front desk said to me that I must pay $15. I said, "What! I'm here with my friend who invited me, that's all. I'm not going to pay; it's not right. I'm here only to keep my friend company. I'm a bodybuilder and have my own workouts." He changed just like that and wrote me out a pass.

My attitude did this. It has taken me a long way and will do the same for you. Stand up confident and secure in what you believe is fair and right. But be sure to do so without arrogance.

The success you achieve depends on a successful relationship with others. People are that important. When you treat people fairly and lovingly, you do not know how it will work out, but it will. You will find that people do things for you, although it may be years before you recognize how a good deed returned to bless you.

People go out of their way to help me wherever I go, like eagerly finding things for me in the grocery store. Why? Because I always leave my house with a good attitude, never a negative one. If I sense I'm not as positive as I should be, as soon as I get into my car I change it. *I do not have the right to make someone else's life miserable.* It abundantly pays off for me.

Relationship and attitude are like brother and sister. A right attitude creates a pathway for people to like you and for you to like them. You seek to understand them and love follows.

Life flows abundantly from a sympathetic, kind, and loving regard for others.

What do I do with negative people?

People often ask, "What do I do with negative people?" If they work for me, it won't be for long before they're out the door. I refuse to allow someone's negativity to pull down what I'm building up. Why would you have someone in your business—or your life—who takes away from it?

I was in New York with my daughter, Adriana, who has a fashion production company. I watched how an employee who, with total control, successfully dealt with 100 people each day. Her standout energy, determination, perfection, and quality of working with others throughout the day awed me. I did not hear one employee say anything bad about her or her work. Everyone respected her.

I asked my daughter, "How do you find employees like her?" She said, "Mom, I tell them how I run my business: I will not tolerate negativity."

Some time later, I asked Adriana how Lydia was doing, another employee I had met. "I just let her go because she was no longer good for the company." Adriana had developed the ability to know that Lydia did not fit, and the strength of character to let her go.

Your life is your greatest business. You are its CEO. Why would you allow in people who drain you with a negative attitude, who criticize and tell you what's wrong with you? Why would you listen to them? No, just get rid of them.

But what if it's my mom, dad, or husband? Good question. I'm kind and patient with my mom and never tell her how she makes me feel. It would only make her feel bad and not help her. I simply arrange with my brother to pick her up after 30 minutes and bring her back to his house. This applies to anyone. I learned that when you're with someone, *you* decide when to leave.

We each have a deep well of experience to draw from. Why would you think something that has happened over and over is going to change without you doing something? It's up to you. You're in control— if you take it.

But do it lovingly. You don't have to be offensive or mean-spirited: it's not good for you or the other person. Be healthy in the way you think and talk.

Remove toxic people from your life

You become bitter if you listen to the negativity of people living miserable, unfulfilled lives of sadness. They mind everyone else's business and judge them because they don't have a real life of their own to keep them busy. And certainly don't allow yourself to believe them. Avoid their company.

You are given a finite supply of energy and your task is to allocate that energy to the higher purposes of your existence. This means that you cannot waste that precious energy by becoming involved with people's dramas, which will divert you from your purpose. Your interactions with others will either bring you closer to your purpose or send you further away.

You will not achieve much in life if you waste your energy with people who drain you. You must stay focused on your purpose. You have only so much energy for the day. I love the analogy of the $100 bill. You have in your energy account $100 worth of energy for the week. You spent $5 for this and $10 on that, and if you're not careful, you run out of money by the weekend. And so it is with energy.

Because your energy has a limit for each day, decide how you will use it. Will you spend time with a "friend" who drains you? Will you allow someone to have coffee with you and all she does is talk, talk, talk, and doesn't listen? I know; it's happened to me, but not anymore. There are some people who should not be parked on the front road of your life. You need clarity of purpose to recognize this.

The other day a gentlemen approached me at the gym and wanted to socialize, interrupting my workout. I go to the gym to work out, not to socialize. After he finished with his comments I said, "Sorry, but I am competing next week and need to stay focused on my workout." He apologized and moved on to someone else to continue chatting. I have an investment of time and a schedule to do it in.

I remember another day when someone began talking to me, wanting to chat, again siphoning time from my workout. I said, *with kindness*, "I must prepare for my trainer and can no longer talk with you." No problem; she got it and didn't feel bad. That's wisdom from a heart of loving kindness.

Develop an attitude that respects your time and energy. If you don't respect it, others will not. And do the same with others; respect their time. Be sure they are up to talking or spending time with you. Why not ask them if it's a good time to talk when you call someone? Simple.

You have decisions to make. Because you have a purpose, you refuse to squander your life-force and your time. *Carpe Diem. Carpe Momentum* (seize the day; seize the moment).

• • •

I'll conclude this foundational section for transforming your life with a truth demonstrated in the life of Victor Frankel. *Attitude* not only enabled him to survive Auschwitz during World War II but he also became a man in control of his destiny.

Creating your dream

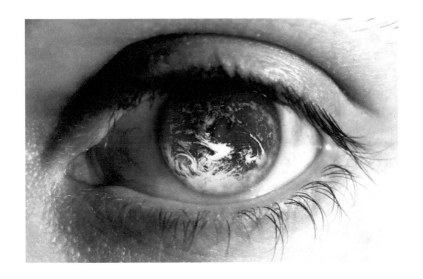

Visualization

Visualization is also called guided imagery, mental rehearsal, meditation, and a variety of other things. No matter the term, the basic techniques and concepts are the same. It is Visualization; it is the process of making something visible to the eye of the mind.

In order to imagine you first need a dream, a picture or a feeling that entices you to dream about it, whatever your circumstances and whether or not it seems doable. Anything is possible in your mind.

In college each evening, after finishing my training in track and field, I would lie down on the grass, close my eyes, and imagine my ideal future. I experienced the feelings and saw the details of me graduating.

Guided imagery, visualization, mental rehearsal, or other such techniques can maximize the efficiency and effectiveness of your training. I continue to visualize my bodybuilding competitions. In 2009 I was having problems with my hip and was in constant pain. The only way that I could practice my bodybuilding posing routine was to see myself doing my poses perfectly. I was mentally and emotionally at the event, hearing the crowd cheer me on with shouts of encouragement. I felt the energy or the crowd and saw faces of the judges pleased with my presentation.

I also visualized myself free of pain and my hips perfect. I always claim perfect health as mine! I am happy to say that my hips and health followed this program of visualization, and they remain in perfect shape.

I visualize almost everything. Visualization is a way of life! It is an area of life in which you have complete control over a successful outcome. With mental rehearsal, minds and bodies become trained to actually perform the skill imagined.

Visualization step by step

The first step I discovered was to calm myself, relax, and then visualize my ideal self. Find that special place and time where you can relax, close your eyes, and let your imagination take you to that special place where dreams becomes reality.

The duration of your visualization depends on how long you can hold the mental picture. Hold it for as long as it feels right. You'll get a sense of this as you practice.

The second step I discovered was that the best time to do your visualization is early morning or late evening. I prefer morning, the time of creation and new beginnings, fertile ground for seeding the new you. Early morning allows you the whole day to carry the new you in your mind. You will unconsciously make the day-to-day decisions that bring you closer to your morning vision. For those who are "evening people," it will reap the same harvest.

Visualization is one key to personal success. It nurtures your self-respect and honors who you are. Remain faithful to the habits that keep you aligned with your true self and the world around you.

The third step I discovered was to use *all* my senses to really see places, people, and things, experience the smells, touch the objects and people, hear the sounds—and to savor the new life visualized before me.

The fourth step I discovered was to feel the emotions of being there and doing what I wanted to do; feeling the excitement of the unknown, the new language, and the new adventure!

The fifth step I discovered is that energy emanates from this invisible reality, waiting to manifest in a natural, stress free way through commitment and *action*! Repeated imagery builds the confidence that comes from experience. It also creates heightened mental awareness and imparts a sense of well-being. These factors in the sports world contribute to an athlete's success. And likewise to *your* success.

The sixth step I discovered is Action! More action! And still more action!

When it comes to action you need to realize that you have been visualizing all your life. For some people visualization pictures their desires vividly; others verbalize detailed word pictures and affirmations.

You visualized as a child what you wanted for Christmas. You thought about it. You talked about it. You asked for it. And you *felt* the feelings of having your favorite gift along with seeing it.

The only difference now is that you use this powerful technique not occasionally but every day to design and create your present reality.

• • •

With this powerful tool you create and control successful performance in all areas of your life.

Visualization has no limitations. You can visualize your ideal body. You can visualize your ideal financial situation, loving relationships, a rewarding career, harmony and balance in your life—a together person.

A very useful tool to aid your visualization is what I call a Treasure Map. You materialize your visualization into the physical world via pictures or drawings on a poster board. These images depict what you want to materialize. The representation and creation of yourself mentally on a treasure map is an exciting and fun activity. You think to yourself, *My God, I have really accomplished something*, as you watch your thoughts morph into action and take form in the physical world; you can touch it, see it, feel it.

One powerful use of the Treasure Map is the feelings and desires that emanate from these pictures. The more powerful the feelings, the faster you will take action. Your creative mind, both subconscious and superconscious, will supply the inspiration, ideas, and motivation.

As a bodybuilder I made a Treasure Map with the poses of bodybuilders I wanted to emulate. I would also watch videos to learn how to pose, which I continue to do. I have won the best female poser award in many competitions. Mentally painting a crisp picture of what you want to achieve is a powerful technique.

So get to work and continue to visualize, but with the difference that you are now doing it consciously and with purpose. You now know that if you can imagine it and you are determined to ride in that direction, then nothing outside you can stop you from reaching your destination. Happy trails to you!

Ready, Set, Action

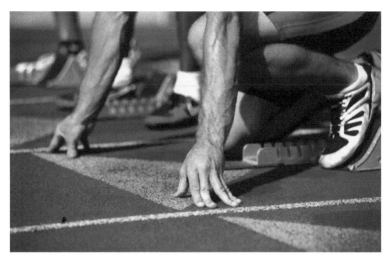

Ready means that you are in a suitable state for an activity. You are prepared mentally and emotionally, ready for action. The foundation of this state of readiness is the belief in your vision and your determination to realize it.

Your vision inspires the ideals and thoughts that prepare you physically, mentally, and spiritually to pursue your God-given talent. Belief provides the energy and creativity that activates your dream. Determination is the engine that drives you to act.

The connection of faith to spirit allows you to hear your inner voice saying, *This is the way, walk in it*. It often expresses through intuition. How do you recognize that "Voice?" You will discover, as you obey your inner voice, that over time it becomes easier to hear and act on it. Things will go perfectly and that builds confidence in the leadings of your spirit. There is then a moment in your life when spirit takes over. Even if you try not to listen and continue to do things your way, the spirit will nag you in a nice way that will make you smile and say, "Okay! I will obey." You will begin to live on a different plane of reality.

Wherever spirit directs, whether or not you personally like it, go there! Let me emphasize *personally like it.* Learn to distinguish between the human you and the divine you.

When spirit leads, you will see each experience and every circumstance as preparing you for the adventure ahead. Be patient while action works its magic as you follow the spirit.

Become aware that many people think they know what is best for you. If you have the clarity of that inner guidance, it will be easy to walk gently away from their unsolicited ideas about your destiny. Having this connection frees you to follow your own way. You confidently express your thoughts and feelings. This quality is the trademark of people who have achieved their dearest goals.

Be persistent. Continue steadfastly in a course of action in spite of difficulty or opposition.

When you connect to your spirit, you hear the inner voice. As an example, I had a burning desire to pursue my higher education because it was the only option for my future.

I would continually visualize and see that reality in my mind. However, for my spirit it was already done! That is when I discovered that we are designed for success. We just need to tune in

After my training in the evening, I would lay down on the beautiful green grass and go at it with my dreams. In one of those visualizations, my inner voice suggested that I reach out and meet with the Minister of Education. Thank God I obeyed!

Here's how my persistence paid off. Meeting with the Minister of Education was not an easy task.

Unknowingly, I had placed myself in an organization where I met people with connections at that level. They told me that the Minister of Education arrives at work at 5 AM. Guess where I was at five o clock that next morning? He would say to me, "Come back tomorrow. Guess where I was the following day?

Finally, he granted me an audience! That is persistence. When you want something with all your heart and might, nothing can stop you. After my meetings with the Minister I did everything the system required me to do to get my financial aid. This process required one year of persistence, passion, determination, and enthusiasm. Giving up was not an option!

It still amazes me that once you decide to do something for your life, the doors open and people and resources appear. This way of doing things began my personal transformation. In a conscious way, I was developing new habits and skills that would support my new lifestyle. It comes down to personal accountability. It is up to me.

Your belief, desire, persistence, and enthusiasm draw into you the magnetic energy that attracts the outworking of your desires, dreams, and goals in the natural world. Your mental and spiritual worlds are real!

The right people

It's thrilling how just the right people show up. They help without dictating how to live your life. Instead they listen and guide you on the path *you* chose, making sure you stay the course, and that you focus on it and not them.

I would ask my teachers for help. They were the only people I knew who had already done what I wanted to do. No one becomes successful without guidance and a helping hand. I also learned to stay away from the naysayers; they will not help you.

One technique that has worked well for me is to select those achievers who inspired and motivate me, and I follow their example. The criterion for me is: Wow! I would love to be like her, or look like her, or have what she has, or do XYZ!

I discovered in college my desire to pursue a Master's degree; my teachers had inspired me; I was so excited. They became my source of information of how to achieve my goal. Surround yourself with these people; they have been there and done it.

I applied this technique to earn my doctoral degree. My mentor was my boss, Dr. Beverly Whitely. I was working at Barry University as an Academic Adviser for the Department of Adult Education. I told her that I I wanted to continue my education. She not only told me how to do it but also mentored me until I graduated. Outstanding person!

Physical Health and Wellness

Prevent the preventable
and cure the curable

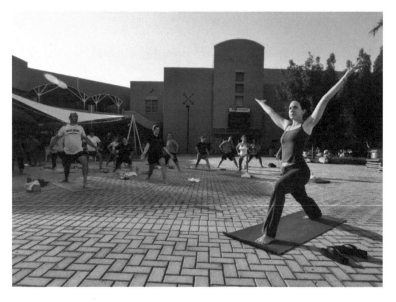

The first wealth is health
Ralph Waldo Emerson

Lifestyle consists of body, mind (thoughts and feelings), and spirit. This section deals with developing skills and habits to heal and preserve a healthy body.

Beauty comes from inside

Be ever mindful of the beautiful body God has given you, and make decisions that keep it that way. Will you eat that seductive doughnut? Or that wholesome apple?

It is essential to keep the beautiful system God has given you in tiptop shape—all your parts: bones, circulatory system, digestive system, muscles, and so on.

You are a Lamborghini, not a junk car. You don't put junk gas in a Lamborghini; you fill it with the best grade. This is why I choose the highest quality food with all natural ingredients and the most effective exercises—the highest grade of whatever touches my body. Don't settle for cheap. *You get what you pay for* is more than a catchy phrase; it's true.

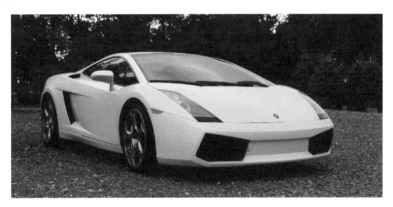

Lamborghini

Skin: the external part of beauty

Want to know how your body is doing inside where you can't see? Look at your skin. It is the largest organ; it reveals the aging process and reflects your internal health. Prevent premature aging by taking care of your skin. Here's how I do it:

- I keep it simple. Less is more. Simplify, simplify, simplify. If in doubt, I don't use it.

- I clean and moisturize my skin with coconut oil every day—my first beauty secret, which I learned from my grandmother. She had the silkiest skin and no wrinkles. She used coconut oil on her whole body and her hair. She died at an age when most people are white-haired—but not her. She would make the coconut oil herself. We children would grate the coconuts and she cooked the oil and strained it. And Pow! there it was, coconut oil lovely and fresh, ready for use.

  As people often do, I strayed from the truth of this simple but powerful secret in favor of what was popular. I spent a lot of money on creams that couldn't touch the benefits of real coconut oil. I finally learned better and now coconut oil is my cleanser and moisturizer. If you want silky healthy skin, get a *pure*[1] coconut oil and use it all the time.

- I never go to bed with makeup on my face; it will age your skin faster than any other factor. A beauty consultant told me that if you go to sleep regularly with makeup on, it will age you 10 years. Not for me!

---

[1] *Pure* coconut oil means processed by the expeller-pressed method with no chemical processing.

- What type of cosmetics should you use? I stay close to nature, meaning as close as possible to how it left the ground, such as pure coconut oil. I refuse to use heavy-duty cleansers with all its chemicals and toxins. Yuck!

Energy has no age

When was the last time you did something you really enjoyed? You loved it so much that time flew by and you couldn't believe it was over? It energizes you, doesn't it? Play, play, and then play! You are never too old to have fun. Playing rejuvenates and energizes not only your body but also your soul. Never disconnect from the child in you.

Set your day right with a morning ritual that vitalizes you. Here's what works for me, after which I can do all I need in the day.

- Wake at 4 AM. Not as difficult as it may sound if you go to bed early and sleep well. But find a time that works for you; that's the key.

- Meditate and pray. Communing with God sets the spiritual foundation for the day. From spirit flows the highest source of your well-being into your mind, and thence into your body.

- I walk three miles and run another three miles. But that's what works for me. If you enjoy walking as an exercise, 30 minutes each day works well. If you are able, walk at a good pace, around three miles an hour.

- Thirty minutes of yoga comes next.

The result? I feel connected, strong, and optimistic, looking forward to what the day brings. Find what brings you this result.

Exercise

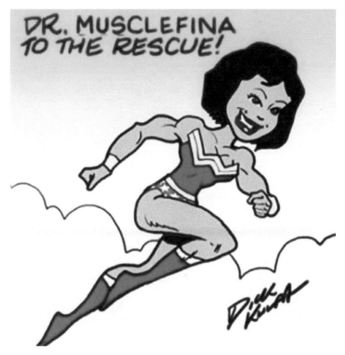

In my philosophy, you eat every day, you breathe every day, and you exercise every day. We are designed to move. The secret of the fountain of youth is not buying the most expensive makeup. You achieve it by exercising. You do not have to wait three weeks to feel good; you feel better right away. Get moving and you will feel great!

One of the best ways to stay young is to develop your muscles. If you don't use it, you lose it because muscles degrade from disuse. Muscles are your largest source of energy. They keep your metabolic system intact, protecting you against metabolic and hormonal decline, obesity, diabetes, and cardiovascular disease. Another reason it's crucial to maintain your muscle mass is the hormones they produce. So many people feel bad because they are hormone deficient, and this is a simple way to increase their production and keep them balanced.

The loss of muscle means loss of energy, a tendency to gain excess weight, vulnerability to disease, and accelerated aging. Get going!

Weightlifting

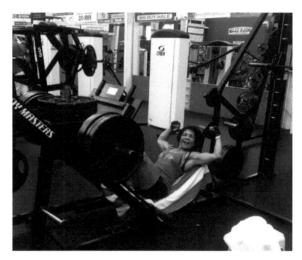

For me, weight lifting is essential to successful aging. I do two hours of weight training daily. It suits me because I'm a bodybuilder (at least for now; I find that I change my focus every ten years or so). For those without such a physical focus, less lengthy and intensive exercise will do fine.

If you don't want to say with dismay, *How haggard I've become*, change your way of thinking. Activity that follows your thinking ensures that your muscles remain strong, that your bones retain their density, that your skin stays beautiful, that your joints remain flexible. Even if you now see yourself decrepit, that can and will change. ☺

Yoga

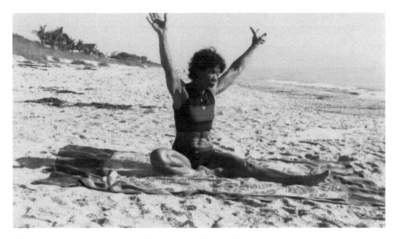

Yoga was a natural transition from being a gymnast. It demands discipline, which resonated with me. It also encourages simple living and high thinking.

Yoga's discipline integrates body, mind, and spirit. I have always believed that to be healthy you need to cultivate your mind, your body, and your beautiful spirit. As the scriptures say, your body is the temple of the Holy Spirit. It needs right food, right exercise, right breathing, right relaxation—and thinking positively, the key to happiness.

To keep my body in ideal health, after my morning walk and run, I do 30 minutes of Yoga. It prevents injuries and keeps my whole body flexible and in balance.

The benefits of Yoga are profound. I believe in it so much that I traveled to Calcutta, India where I became certified in Yoga therapies.

What type of exercise is best?

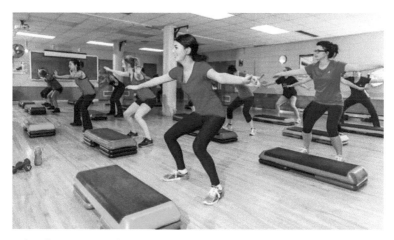

The best exercise is the one you love because you will stick to it and won't quit. It will not work if you don't enjoy it. Ideally choose one where you can't wait to get up in the morning and get going: walk, bike, swim—whatever works for you. Everyone's body is unique and requires exercises suited to it. The secret is to discover what you love and your body feels natural doing.

I have discovered those activities that I love and my body appreciates. I particularly like yoga. It keeps your body flexible and limber at any age, especially for those who can't or do not want to walk, run, or exercise strenuously.

How much should you exercise?

As much as you want. If you finish your program and feel it is enough, then it is enough. Once you really enjoy exercising, your body will tell you how much. Time is not as important as learning to read your body. For example, after you finish walking and feel like going on, do so.

I tell my clients who do not exercise to begin with 10 minutes. I know in a week they'll be doing 15 minutes, then

20, and progressively more until it's the right amount of time for them. One of my clients began working with me as a heavy woman. It wasn't long before she would say at our counseling sessions, "I can't wait to finish our appointment so I can walk."

Don't cut short the things you love. What a shame when you're having a good time and all those thoughts crop up that you need to do this, go here, see that person. Learn to release these thoughts. Thank them but send them on their way. There is a time for them, but not during your exercise! Dedicate the best part of your day to it.

After I finish my exercise I have plenty of time for everything else; it's wonderful how it happens. When you take care of what's important, everything unfolds in a beautiful and timely manner. Life is on your side and it opens up the way in which you should go. You don't have to worry about it.

Manage your stress

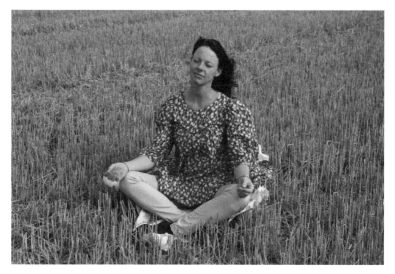

Researchers know the stress we face over our lifetime and how well we cope with it as one of the most significant factors for predicting how well we age.

Successful agers know the value of quiet, restful, and contemplative time. Out-of-control stress accelerates aging. While it's crucial to deal with such stress—and there are many ways to do so—how much better it is to prevent it. How to do so? *Each day* rest, relax, and refresh, which are essential for outstanding performance—bodybuilding for me, but whatever delights and energizes you.

How well you cope with stress is determined largely by following what comes earlier in the book. For example, taking your daily walk while admiring the skies, taking in the trees, gazing at a lovely boat in the river, delighting at the dolphins swimming. Your mind immediately changes direction; no longer are you focused and plagued by ugly things.

Let your life embody commitment, responsibility, passion, determination, and the heartfelt belief that you are worthy and valued. It is your right to be happy and enjoy every single day. You're not supposed just to get by and suffer. I tell people I don't want to suffer—not me. And neither should you.

A beat-up heart breaks the spirit while a grateful heart wears a smiley face.

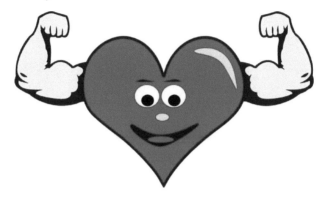

Sleep

Your ability to sleep soundly is an excellent indicator of how well you manage stress and maintain balanced physical, mental, and emotional health—and a spiritual connection.

Start your day by meditating and communing with your spirit. During the day take a siesta if you can and if it works for you. Then get a good night's sleep.

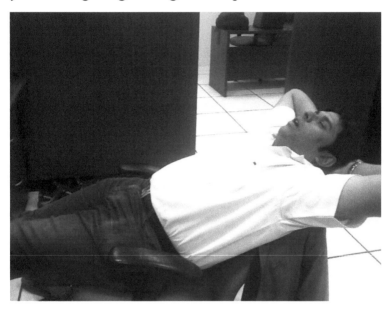

A lot happens when we sleep. On the physical level, for example, human growth hormone, which is part of an extensive repair and restoration effort, is released (also when you exercise). Because I want to stay youthful, slow the aging process, and not pay $1000 for some doctor to put fake hormones in my veins that supposedly keeps me young, I make sure to sleep well.

Your spirit also works during the night doing the restoration work of body-healing, mind-organizing, and soul-forming. That's why after a genuinely good night's rest you awake invigorated, often with ideas for decisions you must make and solutions to problems you must resolve.

Make a ritual before going to sleep. Here's mine: I go to sleep by eight o'clock, winding down by six or seven. I don't watch TV or do any heavy duty stuff. I thank my divine Father for the day and his overcare. Result: I slide into bed with a peaceful and restful mind.

Begin the day with reverence and end the day with reverence. In between have fun.

Nutrition

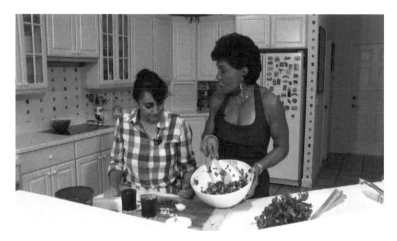

It's very simple. Eat the things that God made, not what man has modified, processed, and chemicalized, which is why people are sick. Whatever has roots—it grows out of the ground—is good for you.

What do I eat? Nutrition, like everything else, must suit your make up. Each person's nutritional profile differs. I coach and encourage my clients is to find which foods work for them: foods that give them energy, foods that keep them healthy, foods that slow down the aging process. It's all possible! If you are determined to be healthy, you will make the time to discover your nutritional blueprint. It is not difficult. Keep a log of what you eat for three weeks and how you feel.

When I began bodybuilding in 2005, I saw everyone eating rice. So I thought, *I'll eat rice too*. Big mistake! Each time I ate rice I felt my blood sugar rise, and I was hungry again in 30 minutes. Hmm, something was wrong. I needed to find an alternative. Lucky for me I discovered sweet potatoes. They keep my blood sugar balanced, and I'm not hungry in an half-hour. But it took paying attention to my body to discover my nutritional plan.

What I eat

I eat oatmeal, sweet potatoes, white potatoes, and meat, eggs, chicken, and fish in moderation. Veggies are my favorites, particularly broccoli, cauliflower, and green beans. Here's an example of a typical day:

- For breakfast, ½ cup of oatmeal.
- Three ounces of steak before I go to the gym.
- After my workout, egg whites with a whole egg.
- For lunch, chicken, broccoli, cauliflower, and sweet potato.
- My last meal (4:30-5:00 PM) is similar, changing the protein to fish. (I don't snack after this meal; I've been eating throughout the day and it's sufficient for my nutritional needs.)
- The oils that work for me are olive, coconut, and avocado oil—naturally processed without heat or solvents.

Keep in mind that I burn a lot of calories bodybuilding, so you won't need as many. And a reminder: what works for me may not work for you. As I did, you must discover what makes your body feel first-rate. Once you find the formula for the foods that your body loves, why change? Stay with what works. It's simple.

Medical care

This is a bold statement: If you're feeling good, there is no need to go to the doctor. It may sound foolish because doctors tell you that you *must* have regular checkups.

I don't go to doctors because I have no concerns about my body. I feel happy, I feel good, I have energy. When people ask me if I go to the doctor, I tell them, "No, I manage my own health. Don't I know my body better than anyone else?" You go to a doctor and he or she gives you an opinion, and then another one tells you something different. They drive you nuts. Prevent what's preventable and cure what's curable.

Take charge of your own health. Why would you put your well-being in someone else's hands? Because it's too much effort to think about? Because you don't want to walk five minutes and you drive instead? Because it's easier to buy a TV dinner with 500 mg of salt in one bite? (Okay, I'm exaggerating, but you get the idea.)

Make time to plan your health. People spend more time preparing for a vacation than planning their health.

Fortunately, it's not too late for *anyone*. It's incredible how the body heals itself. Take control with passion. Become accountable and take responsibility for your own health instead of taking the easy way and letting a doctor do it for you. Spend the time to learn and understand your body and how to keep it in tiptop shape. Otherwise, it won't work.

Epigenetics

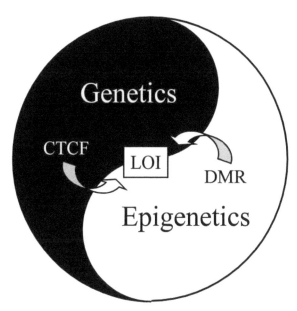

What ages you is your lifestyle. Genetics no longer plays the role we once thought. Because your father had a heart attack doesn't mean you will too. We can change how genes express themselves, either for good or for bad. This is a new way; science is on our side. It's up to you. Believe you have a choice and do something knowing this.

Genes appear to be limited to biology, but how you live determines how they affect your body. It's not preordained that the genetic inclination to cancer you were born with must express itself. It doesn't have to be so! You have power! I want people to deeply connect and know they are neither helpless nor victims. No, they are conquerors! They can master their bodies and control their minds and principle their emotions.

Epigenetics empowers you to no longer be a victim. But it requires you to answer with determined commitment the question Jesus asked the sick person: *Do you* want *to be well?*

Yes? Then you *must* change your lifestyle. This means avoid as much as you can toxins in the food you eat, the air you breathe, the water you drink, the cleaners you clean with, the thoughts you think, the feelings you entertain, the people who pollute you—everything! It's not a small commitment to do this.

Some people prefer to remain victims and stay sick, in not only their bodies but also their minds and emotions. Emotions tell you it's too much effort to be well. I want to, but it's too hard. To become powerful takes guts, courage, discipline, self-control, and a lot of effort. Do the work now to live an energized life forever.

Energy underlies everything. It is neither good nor bad; it just is. Become one with your energy in whatever you do, whether it's washing the dishes or cleaning your house. This means living in the moment so your mind is not all over the place and you can't focus on what's right in front of you. It's incredible how time flies when you are fully connected with what you are doing and go with its flow. You become timeless. Don't ask me what day it is; I'm timeless.

• • •

I'll finish the section by repeating the place of attitude in building your physical body. It comes first. Without a good and right attitude effort merely becomes exercise.

Spiritually Forever Young

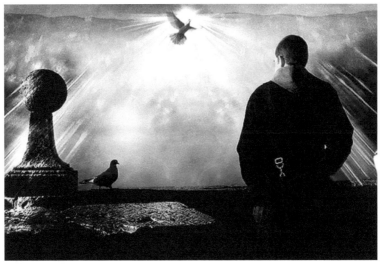

Spirit brings to pass what you believe

The goal

Spirit governs all that is beneath it: body, mind, and emotions. Grow your spiritual life to achieve a powerful body, creative mind, and mature emotions. Cultivate *equally* your body, mind, emotions, and spirit. It's how you become well-balanced and less likely to be thrown by unexpected events that come your way.

The word "disease" is comprised of two parts: dis + ease, your body lacking ease or being *ill* at ease. Physical disease stems from a mind disturbed, emotions unsettled, and a spirit neglected. Your body reflects not only its intelligent care, but also the state of your mind, and spirit. Do not think you can heal your body and maximize its strength without also attending to the development of morals, sociability (getting along with others), emotional maturity, and a spiritual life. And pervading these components of selfhood is a loving, compassionate desire to help others.

Develop a higher point of view. Have the attitude that every day you are growing and perfecting because God is working through you, and you are doing it for his pleasure and delight. Seeing things from on high makes sense of everything.

You are the co-creator with eternity of your destiny. I am content to let life unfold my destiny in its time, helping it by living each day to its fullest.

The spiritual dimension of your life

Your systems—body, mind, and spirit—work together, unified by personality, to develop you as a whole person. We are a blend of material, mental, and spiritual energies. People often neglect the spiritual side of their lives. The result? They lack spiritual energy. Why is this important? It is from spirit that energy flows into your mind and body.

The physical body is the foundation on which rests spiritual consciousness with its spiritual energy. If it is sick and weak, your body limits you in every way. That's why staying healthy is so important.

Your body is a beautiful machine. Deciding that developing spirit is not important is like driving an automobile with eight cylinders, but is running on only four. You think being unable to accelerate faster or climb steep hills is a problem with the car. You don't realize there are four cylinders doing nothing and performance could be so much better.

When you function only on the levels of mind and body, you don't know what you're missing and what you can become. Picture the Lamborghini previously discussed. Enrich your spiritual life to make this your car in spirit. Zoom!

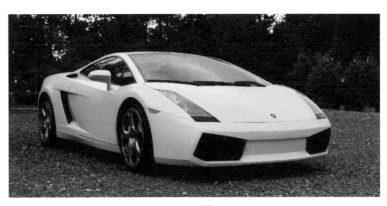

Connecting with your Higher Power

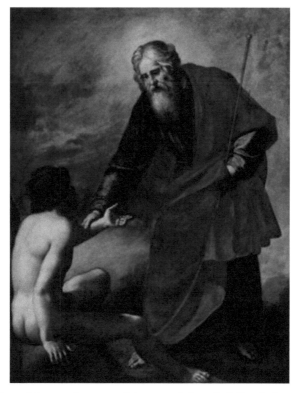

God has blessed me with a spiritual life. I have always believed and trusted him. I would not have my wonderful life if it weren't for my faith and confidence in my heavenly Father.

As long as I can remember I have felt something larger and greater than myself. I didn't know what it was, but how I loved the sense of peace, confidence, and security that embraced me.

My grandmother was a woman of God. She would take us to the Holy Week procession that showed Jesus crucified on the cross. It made an overwhelming impact on my spiritual life. He became my source of hope, belief, confidence, and trust.

As a teenager I would argue with my mom, and she would afterward find me at church kneeling and praying. God was my go-to person. I would tell him about my fears, problems, dreams, and desires. I have been guided always about what to do and what path to take. It remains true to this day that whatever I need is provided. All my heart's desires have been fulfilled and more. All is well with my soul.

My clients tell me about similar blessings. The joy is so tangible that it remains in your heart and mind. The grace and blessings of the Lord must be experienced. How can you describe the flavor of mangos?

I believe Jesus when he said, "Be perfect, even as your heavenly Father is perfect." I daily work and walk fearlessly towards the goal of holiness and perfection he set for me.

I encourage my clients to cultivate a relationship with the divine presence in their lives. It makes the journey of life flow. It becomes enjoyable—even fun. Life is so much easier when you connect with your spirit, when you live by the highest principles and values you can perceive, when you trust your spirit who knows all—what to do, where to go, what to say.

Stay connected to remove stress

I make it a point to be in God's presence throughout the day. I thank him for everything I do! I ask him to guide my steps and to cleanse my heart and my thoughts. I reflect on what is of good report; and when my mind wanders, I bring it back to what is good.

I believe God's promises to me. I see them materialize, although in his time, not mine. Because I walk in faith, I know that all things work to my good. So I don't stress out; I don't worry; I have this sense that all is going well and is as it should be.

Stress disconnects us from our spirit. And we remain disconnected because we don't take the time and make the effort to rest, release, and refresh. When we keep going at the rhythm and tempo of craziness, it's not possible to connect with our higher power. The things of the world wrap you up: career, children, bills—it's never-ending.

Catch-22: You cannot see the light when in turmoil. It often requires being wacked enough times that you finally recognize your life is not working; there must be a better way! Then—it seems miraculous—you reconnect with your life within, whether from a walk by the ocean, a vacation in the mountains, or being quiet in your room. You *finally* take a time-out.

People get in trouble when they hear the prompting of spirit—the inner voice, intuition—and they don't follow it. Life brings what you need and tells you what to do. Be proactive and ask, "Tell me what to do today." Then listen for the prompting of your spirit and do it. It's that simple.

Your Divine Parent

It may help to think of spirit as your Divine Parent, for truly he is the most loving and wise Father you can imagine. No longer say, "I don't have time; gotta run." Rather, make it a priority to welcome his presence.

Your spirit can then call you into relaxation, reflection, and connection with the higher part of yourself. you're in trouble until you learn to listen to that still-small-voice and no longer shut it out. My aim is to *never* be in trouble. Anxiety does not touch me when I listen. Then, whatever happens, I have the strength of spirit; it shows me the way and lifts me through it. I have clarity of what is happening, which enables me to deal with it—illness, broken heart, whatever it is.

Prayer

From experience I have learned that an answer to a prayer comes from developing a close relationship with God, from knowing him. The greater your intimacy with God the faster your prayers get answered. Some of my prayers are answered in minutes! It is surreal. You need something and it shows up.

Think of prayer as just having a little talk with your Father.

Talking with your Divine Father shows a familiarity, which is important to cultivate. Someone I know begins his day by crawling onto the lap of his Father, hugging him, and being lovingly embraced in return. No matter what the situation, learn to share your inner life with God, your sympathetic and wise Parent. When in such communion, you will find the answers you need and the direction you should take. Attuning to your spirit *each* day creates a foundation for your day.

Deeply reflect on what's important to you. When you persistently think about something, you're meditating on it, contemplating it, and then it comes to pass in your life.

When you focus your prayers on positive things, things that are loving and constructive, they keep your soul clean.

The answer to prayer I most treasure is each day feeling grateful and blessed! I feel loved and secure. With his loving support I can do anything.

Exercise your spirit

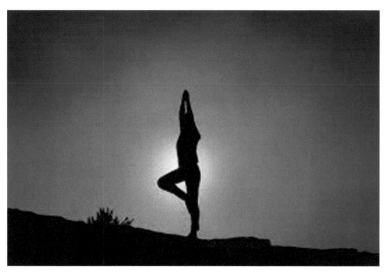

You must nurture a relationship with your spirit the same way you attend to your physical body by eating, sleeping well, and exercising enough. What can you do to align your physical body with your spirit, who lives in an attitude of agelessness that you may also feel ageless?

Think of spirit as a muscle. As you work on that spirit muscle and develop it, there comes a moment when you surrender your self-will to its all-knowing divine will. You're no longer fighting circumstances or anyone. It doesn't mean I don't care about what I'm doing. I do care, but I have a clear picture of why I'm here and how what I'm doing fits into it. Those around me may not support it, believe it, even oppose it, but I know! My spirit guides and tells me what to do. The key is that I obey!

You need to make the time to nurture your spirit connection, like when the doctor says you you need to exercise, walk, and eat better. Same with strengthening your spirit connection. If I don't work on my spiritual life, it's like not working on my muscles, and I'll be falling down with flabby muscles by the time I'm 60. And so it is with developing a relationship with your indwelling spirit guide.

While the external body does deteriorate physically, spirit does not age. You becomes more and more vigorous and creative as you nurture it. The physical body reflects the youthfulness of its spirit. Want a body lovely to behold as you grow older? Simple, connect with your ageless spirit.

You must include a spirit plan to age successfully. It's part of the daily routine. You look at people successful in aging and watch how they care for their spirit. You can't eliminate or ignore this crucial part of aging. It is integral to the process. Running and eating right alone will not do it; you must include your spirit.

People are hungry for spirituality. When I work with people and they mention something about their spirit, I begin talking about it. If they don't bring it, then I do. I include spirit in the life-plan I set up for my clients: what to eat, how to exercise, when to rest, and the importance of meditating (connecting with spirit) before sleeping at night and after rising in the morning. This prepares your spirit for the whole day. Begin the day with spirit and end your day with spirit. Then everything between takes care of itself.

Like yourself

Think of spirit in a personal way, for it is truer than you can imagine. Your heavenly Father loves and approves of you as you are. You are his child. A love-trust relationship with our Creator-Parent is built into us. It's up to us if we'll open ourselves to his loving kindness, patience, and compassion.

Why is it so difficult to believe he is your real Father and live knowing you are okay? No, it's more than okay, much more. From a child we suffer from mistrust, suspicion, and fear—often so subtle that we don't recognize it as an adult. Mistrust is the fabric of our culture; it has imprinted upon our consciousness. It corrupts our relationship with our Creator and with one another. That's why marriages fail and partnerships break up.

Knowing this, work to overcome a false sense of unworthiness. You do this by recognizing and accepting the truth that our value lies in being a child of our loving Father, not what we do well or badly.

You learn who you are by spending time with yourself. So be sure to carve out enough time. The result? How wonderful when you can say, *I like myself.*

Energy

Energy doesn't have an age; it's not 100 years old. My spirit and my energy are one. They are ageless and timeless, and therefore I am ageless because I have energy.

What moves me is the energy of my spirit. People ask me how I have so much energy. They don't know that I spend time developing my spirit the same way I develop my muscles. I work on it every single day!

The first thing I do when I get up is work on my spirit; then I work on my body. *Spiritual strength is more important than physical strength.* You can move things with your spirit. Have you not heard of an incident similar to this woman who saw a kid crushed by a car and she lifted the car! Where did that strength come from? It's not from going to the gym. It came from spirit. That might be the moment of awakening for her: "My God! I didn't know I had that!"

If you don't work on your spirit, you will still have some energy; perhaps 5% instead of 100%. And you wonder why you don't have energy. My energy doesn't come from my flesh, my body; it comes from my spirit.

Afterword

I received a standing ovation at a competition. While it was gratifying to see everyone's appreciation so enthusiastically expressed, more satisfying was knowing what my life portrays got through. Namely, you can remake yourself and be whoever you want to be. That's what this book is intended to inspire.

Judges at competitions point me out to others because my delight and enthusiasm exemplify what a bodybuilder needs. Nonetheless, I ask the judges, "What can I do to get better?" They exclaim, "What can you say! You inspire us. Keep doing what you are doing; you have the formula." And so can each of us have the formula.

Your life is comprised of energy: physical, mental, and spiritual. From it life-force proceeds, whether positive or negative. The more you align with your life's purpose—your dream and your hope—the more forcefully does your life speak louder than words. You become your dream.

Life is too short to do things you don't like. Be passionate; it's what life is about. Why are you here? When your purpose is clear, you do all with gusto. While the ultimate reason for your life does not change, the form in which it expresses itself does. Be flexible and go with the flow.

Here I am, a 70-year-old woman (I don't like the sound of that; I'm 70 years young!), but with a youthful vitality and physical health that is timeless. If I can do it, so can you. Let it be so in your life.

What my clients have to say

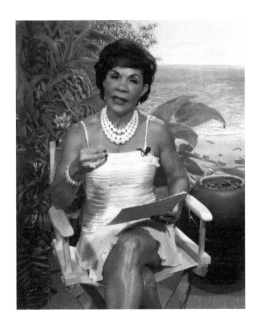

I thought to share how my clients have changed and wrote new chapters in their lives by applying the principles I put into this book. Let them encourage and inspire you to write your own chapter. If you do, I'd love to hear how you did it. Would you please send your story to me at DrJosefina@att.net.

Took control of my food intake

I was frustrated with my weight gain and my inability to get back on track with many things in my life. I had been working over a hundred hours a week and found it nearly impossible to get control of my food intake at work. I told Dr. Josefina the challenges I was facing and that I needed accountability since I was unable to get the motivation I needed to lose fifteen to twenty pounds. My clothes were getting tight on me and I was not feeling good about the way I looked. I was also not able to get enough energy and motivation to start back at the gym or to return to my Zumba classes.

Dr. Josefina worked with me continuously over the course of ten weeks, and I started to set goals and make significant changes in my life. I lost 15 pounds within the ten weeks and worked on many life goals as well. With her instruction I learned a lot about nutrition and which foods worked to make my weight loss more successful and which ones helped to build lean muscle. At her suggestion I hired a personal trainer and started working with weights to build muscle and improve body tone. I lost inches almost immediately. In fact, I lost eleven inches off my measurements after losing only five pounds.

I used the tools that Dr. Josefina provided for me and worked on saying affirmations and taking time to meditate once again. My spiritual life had been neglected along with other things in my life. I realized more than ever that my life was out of balance. With Josefina's help I was able to get back on track.

I also started setting goals for the future. One goal was to get a teaching certificate. I had a bachelor's degree and felt that it would be beneficial to go one step further and apply to

IPE program where individuals with a bachelor's degree in something other than education can get certified to teach in Florida. I was accepted to the program at Indian River State College and plan to start classes in the fall. I can take classes and keep working my present job because many of the classes are online. I also set new goals for significant relationships in my life, along with setting boundaries. I also plan to add adventure to my life with a photo shoot where I can get visual proof for the world and myself that anyone can make positive changes no matter what the age. Another of my new goals is a trip to Paris in September.

Dr. Josefina is readily available via text or email to her students. She is supportive in the challenges you face. She has numerous YouTube videos which helped and motivated me.

I have thoroughly enjoyed having her as my coach. She is such a role model because she lives the principles she teaches. If I could channel one thing from Dr. Josefina, it would be the look of determination that she possesses. She looks at what she wants to create with this fierce and confident look and she then manifests her desires. She has used this technique in her life and I'm using her techniques to manifest all that is important to me in my life. Thanks to Dr. Josefina, I hold my head up a higher and have hope that the present and future will be what I make it.

Michelle Schlefsky

Empowerment

This is to all who want to know the empowerment you can experience with this incredible lady.

I was just beginning to work out again and Josephina happened to be at the gym also working out. We started to chat (we've known each other for 20 years) and she suggested we train together for six weeks while she prepared for a competition. I agreed and we set a time.

When we met for our first workout she handed me her workbook and said, "If you are serious about changing your body and making positive changes in your life, we need to do both external and internal transformation."

This has been my most exciting life change, both mentally and physically. I lost 28 pounds and my attitude has been revitalized. I look forward to each day knowing that the universe, God, and my dearest friend's inspiration, knowledge, and empowerment program have had an incredibly positive impact on my life.

I am now looking forward to my first bodybuilding or figure competition this summer. Never in my wildest dreams would I have ever imagined that would ever happen. To you Josephina I give my thanks and my love and eternal gratefulness.

Micki Weilbaker-Conroy

Expect the best from life

Thanks so much for teaching me to believe and expect the best from life again. Since my husband's death four years ago I was stuck in a rut to say the least. By the end of your class I had regained my positive attitude and started talking about my future, and planning it by writing it down and following my "treasure map."

Before your class I would have thought this was a silly thing to do. Nonetheless, I proceeded to cut out a picture of a pretty new house from a real estate magazine, not knowing where the money would come from. Two days later my son called and says, "Mom, I think you should sell your and dad's house here in Ohio and buy a new house in Florida." I had kept the home in Ohio because my children begged me to do so because their dad had built it. I knew they wanted to keep alive memories of their father. I didn't go against their wishes. God does work in mysterious ways, doesn't he?

I thank you for teaching me that it is okay to dream and to expect those dreams to come true. I have five more things I am hoping for and I fully expect to have them in Gods time. Forever Grateful.

Charlene Jarvis

Bless others by your life

(Author note: I included this letter to encourage you to embrace these principles of change not only for yourself but for others as well. The purpose of living is twofold: 1) Become a whole, unified, loving person 2) that you may uplift and bless others by just being yourself, who you are meant to be.)

Don't know if you remember me but I worked for TV 10 WWCI about 7 or 8 years ago. You crossed my mind today when I was thinking about all the people that influenced my life in one way or another.

Though I have never bought any of your tapes or attended your seminars, just your continual positive attitude around me influenced my life so positively. I am living back in Missouri where I was raised, working for an awesome company and doing exactly what I always wanted to do.

I suppose at this point Josefina, I should say thank you for just being you. May your life continue to brighten others, and I hope your life is blessed for it.

Terry

Josefina's Sayings

My sayings

What you do today should be important; you are exchanging your life for it!

Don't worry about your place in the world. Don't worry about what others think about you. What matters is what you think about them.

It's never too late to reap the benefits of exercising. In fact, the older you are, the more immediate is the benefit.

Healthy optimism acknowledges a problem while it concentrates on its solution.

You are limited only by the size of your dreams.

Do not judge me by my successes, judge me by how many times I fell down and got back up again.

A wise person does his or her best to get the most from a situation because once that opportunity has passed, it may not come again, and you will be left wanting.

Sayings of others that I like

You are never too old to set another goal or to dream a new dream. C.S. Lewis

The secret of getting ahead is getting started. Mark Twain

The only limits in our life are those we impose on ourselves. Bob Proctor

There is a difference between interest and commitment. When you are interested in doing something, you do it only when it is convenient. When you are committed to something, you accept no excuses, only results. (War Memorial Auditorium)

Request from the Author

Thank you for taking the time to read *Vibrant at Any Age*. If you found value in it, please post a review, tell your friends, share online. Give others the opportunity to improve themselves. Word of mouth is an author's best friend and much appreciated.

CPSIA information can be obtained
at www.ICGtesting.com
Printed in the USA
BVHW02n1421191018
530590BV00001B/1/P

* 9 7 8 1 5 3 9 7 6 5 8 0 6 *